THE SUDDENLY SUCCESSFUL STUDENT

*A Parents' and Teachers' Guide
to Behavior and Learning Problems*

How Behavioral Optometry Helps

ELLIS S. EDELMAN, Doctor of Optometry
CONSTANTINE FORKIOTIS, Doctor of Optometry
HAZEL RICHMOND DAWKINS

SUTTER HOUSE

MANUFACTURED IN THE UNITED STATES OF AMERICA

LIBRARY OF CONGRESS CATALOGING IN PUBLICATION DATA

Edelman, Ellis S., 1924–
 The suddenly successful student.

 Bibliography: p.
 1. Vision disorders in children—Handbooks, manuals,
etc. 2. Children—Medical examinations—Handbooks,
manuals, etc. I. Forkiotis, Constantine, 1923– .
II. Dawkins, Hazel H. Richmond, 1937– . III. Title.
RE48.2.C5E34   1985   618.92′0977   85-30343
ISBN 0-915010-34-8

Cover art and design by
C. C. Dawkins, The Writing Team

THE SUDDENLY SUCCESSFUL STUDENT
Designed and produced by
SUTTER HOUSE
P.O. Box 212
Lititz, Pa. 17543

Contents

Preface

Doctors Ellis Edelman and Constantine Forkiotis have specialized in behavioral optometry for many years, painstakingly accumulating the knowledge that has gone into this handbook. To this, Hazel Richmond Dawkins has brought her personal experience. When she was seven, she had an operation to "straighten" an in-turning eye. Within months, the eye was turning out. For the next forty years, Hazel was functionally blind in that eye. During those years, in England, France, Switzerland and America, she was told nothing could be done, although the eye was "healthy."

Imagine, then, her amazement when she was referred to Dr. Edelman and learned that her "blindness" was the result of the brain shutting down input from that eye because it didn't fuse with the input from her other eye. She discovered there was a distinct possibility she could learn to straighten her eye, without surgery, and perhaps recover some of the lost sight and vision. Behavioral optometry was the therapy offered, and in the following months Dr. Ellis Edelman delivered on his promises.

In rapid succession, Hazel's husband and three of their five children consulted with Dr. Edelman and were helped to an extraordinary degree. It was at this point that Hazel realized the need for this handbook and enlisted the collaboration of Drs. Edelman and Forkiotis.

Others, in particular the following, have given their support and advice, for which the authors thank them: Dr. Charles Margach of Southern California College of Optometry; Drs. Elliott Forrest, Irwin Suchoff, Nathan Flax, Harold Solan and Beth Bazin at New York's SUNY; Dr. David Friedel in Tucson; Dr. Lynn Hellerstine in Denver, Drs. Beth Ballinger and Gerry Getman in Newport Beach; Tom Lecoq at OEPF; Charlotte A. Rancilio at AOA; Dr. Martin Kane of COVD; and Dr. Richard Apell and Mary Megargee at the Gesell Institute of Human Development.

Ellis Edelman
Constantine Forkiotis
Hazel Richmond Dawkins

1

A Parents' and Teachers' Guide to Vision Problems

About ten million children under the age of twelve in the United States have vision problems that make it hard for them to cope with home and school.

That's the bad news. It comes from the American Optometric Association (AOA), the nation's leading professional organization devoted to the problems of vision and vision care. The AOA makes an important distinction between vision and sight. "Rarely do these *vision* conditions threaten a child's *sight.*" However, "They do . . . often prevent a child's development into a normal, contributing adult . . . by interfering with learning; inhibiting participation in sports . . . and creating frustration that leads to misbehavior, dropping out of school and even juvenile delinquency."

The Association's warning is clear. It is well documented that youngsters with vision problems usually have difficulties with learning in school. They often have trouble dealing with family and friends. They may become so frustrated by their problems that they retreat into rebellion. They can become dropouts. Suicides. Or, menaces to society.

These youngsters are often given gaudy labels: Juvenile delinquent. Problem child. Slow learner. Dyslexic. Learning disabled. The sad truth is that giving children with vision problems such labels is like jailing them for crimes which they just didn't commit.

The good news is this: in almost every case of a child with a vision problem there is a relatively simple solution. It can be supplied by a doctor of optometry who specializes in "behavioral optometry."

The trick is: recognizing the child with the problem and getting the child to the specialist.

Protect the Children

Parents and teachers need to know the symptoms of vision problems.

They need to know there is a difference between "sight" and "vision." "Sight" is the ability of the eyes to focus clearly; it is one of many skills which make up vision. "Vision," is something bigger and all-embracing. When the various visual skills (sight, focusing, converging, fixation, teaming, etc.) integrate efficiently with that part of the brain called the visual cortex, the result is what we call "vision." In short, vision gives meaning to what the eyes send in.

Sight and vision are not the same. Sight is the ability of the eyes to focus clearly, one of many different skills which make up vision. Vision is something all-embracing. When skills such as converging, fixation and teaming integrate efficiently with the brain's visual cortex, the result is "Vision."

Parents and teachers also need to know that the professionals who treat these broad-based vision problems are doctors of optometry who specialize in a particular branch of optometry, "behavioral optometry," sometimes called "functional" or "developmental" optometry.

Their Eyesight May Be Good
But Their Vision May Be Terrible

As a parent or a teacher, you must be able to make this distinction. Most children have healthy eyes. They can score an easy 20/20 on the eyecharts. Even if one eye is a little near- or farsighted and the other eye is not. That is "sight."

"Vision," however, is another thing. If, for instance, one eye is a little farsighted and the other eye is a little nearsighted, they are not able to work together as a team. The message they send to the brain is confusing. One eye delivers one message to the brain, the other eye delivers another.

To a child, this is like being told by a father to do one thing and by the mother to do another. The messages are contradictory. So, the child is faced with a dilemma. Which parent — which eye — does it heed?

When a child's brain is confused by contradictory messages from the eyes, the body becomes a battleground. Under the most extreme circumstances, the brain makes one of several choices. The two discussed here are radical decisions: (1) The brain stops accepting messages from one eye; (2) The brain alternates reception from one eye to the other, a process which slows understanding and creates confusion.

This failure of the eyes to work together as a team is called, appropriately enough, "lack of teaming." A teacher can expect to find symptoms of it in about 5 percent of a classroom's pupils. Once discovered, the child should be examined by a doctor of optometry who specializes in behavioral optometric vision care.

Behavioral Optometry is primarily a preventive health therapy.

However, lack of teaming is only one of a number of vision problems that can affect learning and behavior.

Spotting the symptoms of such vision problems is a challenge for parents and teachers.

2

Does This Remind You of Someone You Know?

James   He's in 3rd grade. He's obviously bright. But, Jimmy can't read as well as his sister in 1st grade.

Sharon   She's a brat, according to her family. Won't cooperate. Won't do as she's asked. Has temper tantrums. Cries a lot. She's 10.

Max   He's 15. He's surly, unfriendly. Doesn't communicate with family or schoolmates. He's on his way to being a dropout. Yet, he's not dumb because he can repeat every commercial he's ever heard on TV.

Kevin   He's 17, tall, strong and handsome. Yet, he's never been able to be active in any team sport. He gets violently car sick, can't watch TV or do homework without getting a headache.

Sally   Everybody knows she's brilliant because she reads incessantly, anything and everything. But, she does poorly in school and tests show this 13-year-old does not understand a lot of what she reads. That came as a surprise to her parents.

Every teacher and many parents will recognize such behavior problems. Roughly 10 percent of children in any classroom will exhibit these or similar difficulties. The youngsters involved will come under the scrutiny of family, teachers, therapists, psychologists and doctors (depending on the symptoms). And these well-meaning people will suggest all kinds of reasons for such problems:

lazy; not trying; hyperactive; emotionally disturbed; learning disabled; delinquent; brain damaged; dyslexic.

Yet, all the individuals mentioned here—from James to Sally—were bright kids who were being victimized *by problems in their vision systems.* One of the most fearful oversights in medicine, education and psychology today is the neglect of children's vision systems. We routinely test for "eyesight" but rarely for "vision imbalances." And, as a result, we allow some of our best and brightest to go down the drain. Every parent and every teacher should know that this doesn't *have to happen.* A classic example is Luci Baines Johnson.

Luci Baines Johnson When she was a teenager, and her father was vice-president of the United States, Luci Johnson was having serious problems with her schoolwork. Her parents, both overachievers, were deeply worried and somewhat embarrassed. Despite their wealth, despite their access to all kinds of learned advice, despite having explored every possible avenue, nothing they had tried had helped.

Then Dr. Janet Travell, President John F. Kennedy's personal physician, suggested that Luci's vision might be at the center of the problem. Luci's parents responded that her eyes had been checked and she had 20/20 sight. Dr. Travell pointed out that Luci's *vision* had not been checked.

As a result, Luci was sent to Dr. Robert Kraskin, a Washington optometrist who specializes in behavioral optometric vision care. A small miracle happened, from Luci's point of view. Once she had completed a program of behavioral optometric care with Dr. Kraskin, she went from academic probation to honor roll. Not only did her schoolwork improve dramatically, she also began to enjoy sports from which her vision imbalance had previously barred her.

The change took time. Before vision care, Luci had experienced headaches and nausea when trying to deal with her schoolwork. But gradually, as her vision system came into better balance, Luci found that her ability to learn grew stronger. Like Luci Johnson, thousands of children and adults who've completed a program of vision care have been able to improve learning and behavior and rid themselves of chronic health problems. Thousands more could benefit from optometric vision care if they knew of it and the optometric specialists who practice this preventive health therapy.

Does This Remind You of Someone? / 11

3

How You May Spot a Vision Imbalance

The kind of learning-and-behavior-related difficulties we are talking about probably will not be uncovered in the typical school eyechart exam or by an examination that is limited to checking eye health and eyesight.

Parents and teachers who note the following symptoms at home or in the classroom should see that the child is given a thorough vision examination by a doctor of optometry who specializes in behavioral optometric vision care.

Directly Observable

- Crossed or turned eyes;
- reddened, watering, burning or itching eyes; encrusted eyelids, frequent styes;
- turning or tilting head to use one eye only; or closing or covering one eye;
- placing head close to book or desk when reading or writing;
- frowning or scowling while reading, writing or doing chalkboard work;
- excessive blinking or rubbing of eyes;
- losing place while reading and using finger or marker to guide eyes;
- spidery, excessively sloppy or hard-to-read handwriting; writing that becomes smaller and crowded or inconsistent in size.

Related to Behavior

- Short attention span for the child's age;
- nervousness, irritability, restlessness or unusual fatigue after visual concentration;

- displaying evidence of developmental or emotional immaturity;
- low frustration level; withdrawn, has difficulty getting along with other children;
- headaches, nausea and dizziness;
- complaints of blurring of vision or of double vision at any time.

Related to Classroom Work

- Saying words aloud or lip reading;
- difficulty remembering what is read;
- omitting, repeating and miscalling words or confusion of similar words;
- persistent word reversals after the second grade;
- difficulty remembering, identifying and reproducing basic geometric forms;
- difficulty following verbal instructions;
- poor eye-hand coordination when copying from chalkboard, throwing or catching a ball, buttoning clothing, tying shoes.

If you notice such symptoms — and they can be subtle — you will be doing the child a lifetime service by calling on the expertise of a behavioral optometrist. In most cases, nonspecialists in the optometric field and ophthalmologists are not equipped to diagnose and treat such learning-and-behavior-related vision problems. Such imbalances of the vision system cannot always be corrected by the commonly prescribed eyeglasses or contact lenses. But, optometric vision care, either lenses alone or in combination with therapy, in the hands of a behavioral optometrist, can be effective in helping the child to acquire the balanced vision skills that are so important to behavior and learning.

All Children Need These Visual Skills
Not All Children Have Them

Many different visual skills are involved in a child learning to cope with living in the complicated worlds of family and school. Young children must learn to understand what's going on around them in order to understand where they fit into things. *Clear sight* is not enough. *Understanding* is the key, and vision plays a major part in understanding.

Growing children must first *learn to read* so that, later, they can *read to learn*. Similarly, the visual skills listed below are needed if youngsters are to succeed in school and in life.

1. Clearness of vision (acuity). This is the ability to see clearly at near and far distances. (Clarity at distance is about the only skill that the usual eyechart examination tests, the Snellen eyechart test that tells you that you have 20/20 acuity or you don't.) Generally, children who have poor distance acuity are nearsighted—that is, do well at reading, less well at sports. The farsighted child tends to have more difficulty reading but, often, does better at sports than the nearsighted youngster.

2. Eye movement skills (fixation ability). This is the ability to point the eyes accurately at an object and to keep the eyes on target whether the object is moving or stationary. Without these skills, you can't follow a moving object clearly, such as a ball in flight. You can't move your eyes smoothly across a line of text on a page. A child can't shift the eyes from a close object to a far one, such as from a notebook to a blackboard in class.

3. Eye focusing skills (accommodation). This is the ability to adjust the focus of the eyes as the distance from the object varies. Copying from the blackboard, for instance, requires constant shifting of focus from far to near and back again. Most children are capable of a large amount of change of focus but fine, *accurate control* breaks down more easily under stress. Excellent eye focusing is a skill common to superior athletes.

4. Eye aiming skills (converging and diverging). This is the ability to turn the eyes inward or outward in looking from objects close up to objects far away and back again. These skills must be closely coordinated with eye focusing skills. Inadequacies in these areas seriously hamper reading ability and athletic performance. Fortunately, these are skills that normally can be enhanced through optometric vision care.

5. Eye teaming skills (binocular fusion). This is the ability to coordinate and align the eyes *precisely* so that the brain can fuse the input it receives from each eye. Even a slight misalignment can cause double vision which, in turn, the brain may try to eliminate by suppressing the use of one eye. In one way or another, the brain will react in a disturbed and defensive manner to confusing signals from the eyes.
6. Eye-hand coordination. This is the ability of the vision system (eye-brain connection) to coordinate the information received through the eyes in order to monitor and direct the hands. This skill is important for learning to write (poor handwriting is often related to poor eye-hand coordination). It is essential to good performance in most sports.
7. Visual form perception. This is the ability to organize images on the printed page into letters and/or words. It is one of the most important skills used in learning to read and is developed through both experience and practice. It can be taught or improved.

4

What Causes Vision Problems?

Most preschool children have good vision. Nevertheless, a small percentage of preschoolers have existing vision-system problems. These can come from illnesses like measles or influenza. High fever, eye or head injury or pregnancy complications may also be factors. The fact is the majority of vision problems go unrecognized until the pressures of schoolwork and study begin to overload the vision system. The sudden impact of "near point" work (reading, writing, drawing, doing numbers, using a computer) causes changes. A tendency to nearsightedness or farsightedness will become more pronounced. An eye may begin to cross or drift. Sight may become blurred or the child may begin to see double.

Most vision imbalances are triggered or aggravated by stress—often, in children, by the visual demands of schoolwork or computer use.

This is a complication for parents and teachers because changes in children's vision usually happen so gradually that few children are aware of them. They assume that everyone sees the same way they do. This can be wildly misleading to the adults in their lives because children may have blurred sight or be seeing double and it will never occur to them to describe the condition.

That's why parents and teachers have to be alert to all the possible vision problems.

The Basic Conditions of Risk

Eye disease. The American Optometric Association tells us that school-age children rarely have serious eye disease. *But,*

AOA explains, there are two types of minor eye infections—blepharitis and styes—that may be indications of imbalances in the vision system. (Blepharitis is an inflammation of the eyelids, which can sometimes be identified by yellowish crusts at the base of the eyelashes.)

Both conditions, which are the results of stress caused by vision imbalances, call for a thorough examination of the vision system by a behavioral, functional or developmental optometrist.

Nearsightedness. What the eye doctor calls "myopia" is commonly called nearsightedness. The AOA tells us that "nearsightedness is the only refractive vision condition that increases significantly in incidence throughout the school years." You can expect to find it in about 3 percent of children between 5 and 9. It increases in incidence to about 8 percent among children 10 to 12. And this rises along with the years of school experience to about 16 percent among teenagers. It's something to be on the lookout for.

Nearsighted individuals can see clearly up close but not at a distance. Watch for these signs:

- students who tend to hold their books closer to their eyes than is normal;
- students who bend their heads down close to the page when they write;
- students who twist their faces into a squint when they are trying to see the blackboard.

Myopia: Preventive Treatment The quick fix most often used for nearsightedness is prescription lenses. Lenses can compensate for and provide good visual acuity. The problem is that these "compensating" lenses usually need periodic changing and strengthening because myopia is progressive.

A more specialized and, in the long run, a more rewarding approach to nearsightedness is behavioral optometry's preventive treatment, in the form of "learning" lenses (in contrast to "compensating" lenses), and vision therapy. Similarly, these and other special methodologies are also used to slow or stop the progression of nearsightedness (myopia control).

What Causes Vision Problems? / 17

Nature designed human eyes primarily for sharp, clear seeing at a distance, the eyes of the hunter, the farmer, the sailor at sea. Our eyes were not designed for the endless stresses put upon them by modern living with our books, TV viewing and computer screens, even high-speed travel.

Today, doctors of optometry who practice behavioral optometric vision care can often prevent, reduce or control the myopia caused by environmental stresses by prescribing "learning" lenses. This type of lens has a mild prescription that reduces the amount of stress on the vision system. Usually, such learning lenses are necessary only for reading and close work.

Farsightedness. This is technically known as hyperopia. The AOA tells us that most school-age children are farsighted—as nature intended them to be. They can usually see well at both distance and near; but, there is a drawback. In most cases, farsighted children have to exert *extra effort* to bring their vision into sharp, clear focus for *both far and near* seeing.

For most such children, this presents no problem. But about 6 percent of children aged 5 to 12 have high degrees of farsightedness and need help to relieve the tension of focusing, especially when using their eyes for close work.

Again, most routine school eyechart exams will not catch such problems. It's up to parents and teachers to recognize the signs. Symptoms of hyperopia include:

- difficulty in concentrating and maintaining a clear focus when reading or doing close work;
- eye or body tension when doing such work;
- muscle fatigue, headaches, nausea, aching or burning eyes after doing close work.
- poor reading ability;
- irritability or nervousness after sustained close-work concentration.

Astigmatism. This is the development of unequal curvature of the cornea. Thus, the light gathered in by the eye is not focused properly. The end result is blurred sight. The AOA notes that only about 3 percent of school-age children have significant amounts of astigmatism; however, this represents an increase from 2 percent for preschoolers. The symptoms of astigmatism are similar to those for other vision disorders and they call for the same action: a thorough vision examination by an optometrist who specializes in behavioral, developmental or functional optometry.

Crossed Eyes and Lazy Eyes. Crossed eyes and "lazy eyes" are two conditions that, while not common, put particular pressures on the children who suffer from them.

Crossed eyes (strabismus) is a condition in which the two eyes do not work together; one eye or the other may turn inward, outward, upward or downward. There are different causes. But the result is poor eye control. Ophthalmologists tend to blame poor eye control on the muscles of the eye and all too frequently advise surgery. The behavioral optometrist believes differently and has a less radical, more promising approach.

The situation occurs because the child's vision system has not learned to make the two eyes work together as a team. In rare cases, paralyzed or partially paralyzed muscles may indeed cause "lazy eye" but such paralysis occurs in only a minute percentage of the population.

It is normal, during the first five or six months, for an infant's eyes to appear crossed or unaligned for brief moments while it is learning to use the eyes together as a team. But, if by the age of 3½ months the misalignment appears to be frequent or long-lasting, or is always with the same eye, the infant should be examined. And the professional most qualified to make this exam is a doctor of behavioral, developmental or functional optometry.

Crossed eyes can also develop at a later stage, as children reach school age. Oddly enough, the development is often so gradual that parents fail to recognize it. They get used to the child's appearance and it seems normal. In this case, the problem may be noticed first by the family doctor or at school.

Crossed Eyes: A Cosmetic and Functional Problem There are two major factors involved in crossed eyes. One, the most obvious, is appearance. Crossed eyes look funny, peculiar, different. And "different" is the last thing your school-age child wants to be.

Two, because of the "difference," crossed eyes can inhibit a child's emotional and social development. They can also cause personality problems by isolating the individual from other youngsters and giving the child a poor self-image.

A child will not usually outgrow crossed eyes. Therefore, parents should seek help as soon as they spot the symptoms.

What Are the Choices? For several decades, the conventional medical treatment for crossed eyes has been surgery. Today, however, the specialists in behavioral optometry strongly recommend *against surgery* particularly in cases which are obviously vision imbalances.

The reasons are several. First, surgery usually does not offer a permanent solution to the problem. In surgery, the eye muscles are cut so that the eyes look straight (if the surgeon has judged it to the precise degree). However, since *no effort is made to teach the eyes how to work together as a team*, the underlying imbalance remains and there is a strong tendency for the eyes to turn again. In many cases, repeated operations are necessary yet there's no guarantee of total success.

In contrast, behavioral optometric vision therapy, which opts not to use surgery or drugs, has a greater success rate in treating crossed or out-turning eyes than does surgery by the ophthalmologists. In fact, because it treats the underlying cause, behavioral optometry may be able to solve the problem because once the eyes learn how to work together as a team, there is less of a tendency for them to turn.

Lazy eye, not lazy child. Amblyopia is often called "lazy eye" and it is a condition in which clear, sharp vision in one eye is lowered or apparently lost and cannot be improved with prescription "compensating" lenses. It affects about 2 percent of children.

The AOA tells us that there are different kinds of lazy eye. The most common type is a side effect or complication stemming from crossed eyes or from a vision condition in which one eye is much more nearsighted or farsighted than the other.

In either of those situations, the two eyes send separate and different messages to the brain, which cannot integrate them. Therefore, as explained before, the brain often *turns off the message from one eye.* Since the ability to see sharply and clearly *is a learned skill*, central visual acuity never develops properly in the eye that the brain has turned off.

The one-eyed vision that results can affect other vision skills, such as the ability to judge distances, although a youngster with a lazy eye will not realize this. Once again, it is left to parents and teachers to identify the condition.

Look for the child who noticeably favors one eye (head-tilting is one clue) or who has a tendency to bump into objects. Since poor vision in one eye does not necessarily mean amblyopia or "lazy eye" (it could be myopia or nearsighted-ness), amblyopia can only be definitely diagnosed by a professional examination. Remember that often the lazy-eyed child becomes one sided in its responses and movements and usually does not develop the concept of opposites; perhaps there will be difficulty in balancing and in sports. Sometimes, certain activities like dancing that require using two sides of the body may be avoided.

Behavioral Optometry believes that near- and far-sightedness and astigmatism are adaptations individuals make so they can perform well. The need for such adaptations may be alleviated when the entire vision system is brought into balance.

Computers: A Recent Threat

The Video Display Terminal of the modern computer is a "growing source of vision complaints," according to the Optometric Extension Program Foundation. (A nonprofit foundation, the OEPF has devoted many years to providing post-doctoral behavioral optometric education and publishing related papers for professionals and the general public.)

A 1985 publication of theirs reports on a variety of evidence that relates vision problems to extended use of VDTs. This evidence is drawn from studies of office workers and from a U.S. Air Force Study of Office Automation; but with computers invading the classroom on a broader and broader scale, parents and teachers should be warned that vision problems will be encountered among children, too.

For instance, in a comparison between workers using VDTs and those who were not, the users experienced nearly double the incidence of irritated eyes, burning eyes, blurred vision and 50 percent more eyestrain. There were related physical complaints, too. Headaches. Aching necks, backs, shoulders and, even, hands.

OEPF also reports a study by Mourant, Lakshmanan and Chantadisai that found "2 hours of VDT usage produced measurable fatigue in the eye accommodation mechanism, as well as an increased blink rate." Because printed material and VDT images differ in quality, VDT "characters are relatively blurred and have small area flicker. Continuous action of the eye lens may be necessary to achieve proper focus on the relatively blurred characters. The small area flicker also necessitates constant adjustment . . . to varying light levels. Close range viewing of VDTs requires *convergence and accommodation of the eyes* for sustained periods of time. The ocular muscles controlling eye movement are likely to be exerted beyond their capacity. . . ."

As we have suggested earlier, visual stress leads to lowered performance. Children react to stress by avoiding work, or doing their work uncomfortably and with lowered comprehension. In some cases, they adapt to stress by becoming nearsighted or suppressing the use of one eye.

Adults must be alert for the symptoms of visual problems especially among youngsters who are now being exposed to concentrated use of computers.

5

Vision-Related Problems
Who Do You Turn to for Help?

Two kinds of doctors specialize in eye care. There is the Doctor of Optometry (O.D.). We know this doctor as an "optometrist." To become an O.D., the optometrist undertakes a rigorous four years of clinical and classroom training at a college of optometry. Typically, this is after four years of earlier college education. A high percentage of students have B.A.'s or higher degrees before they enter a college of optometry.

Optometrists diagnose vision problems and prescribe for their remediation and rehabilitation. They also are educated to detect eye diseases and signs of certain health problems (hypertension, arteriosclerosis, diabetes, etc.); the primary health care they offer is invaluable.*

Ophthalmologists are the other kind of eye-care doctor. Ophthalmologists are medical doctors who specialize in diseases of the eye and eye surgery. Ophthalmologists, too, examine eyes and prescribe lenses. But the ophthalmologist's specialty is treating diseases of the eye with drugs and surgery.

Optometry has many specialty areas. They range from infant care to contact lenses to sports vision. Specialists in these areas can help infants develop healthy vision systems. They can improve the performance of even a champion athlete. Where a learning or behavior problem is related to vision imbalances, behavioral optometry is the specialty to seek out.

---

*The 4-year program at colleges of optometry includes biochemistry, cytology, human anatomy, endocrinology and microbiology, general pharmacology and pathology, sensory and perceptual psychology and clinic work.

Behavioral optometric vision care is the optometric specialty that analyzes and treats the complete vision system.

To recap, here is a vocabulary that can help you sort out the various practitioners and specialists.

1. *Ophthalmologist.* A doctor of medicine whose postgraduate training is in diseases of the eye.
2. *Optometrist.* A doctor of optometry (O.D.) educated to diagnose vision problems and prescribe for their remediation and rehabilitation.
3. *Behavioral Optometrist* (also known as Functional or Developmental Optometrist). An O.D. whose postgraduate training is in behavioral optometric vision care and who examines and treats the entire vision system.
4. *Optician.* A technician who produces and/or dispenses the optical lenses, glasses and other equipment prescribed by optometrists and ophthalmologists.

It is to the optometrist who specializes in behavioral, functional or developmental vision care that parents and teachers should turn when—based on the symptoms described previously—they suspect a child has a vision problem.

Note: Practically speaking, parents should not wait for symptoms. It is simply good health insurance to have a child's vision examined by a behavioral optometrist before age three and again before the child enters school and annually thereafter until adulthood. If this were done, we would find fewer students with learning difficulties and more adults whose lives were happier and more productive.

Let us repeat a warning.

Checking a child's visual acuity on the time-honored Snellen Eyechart, with which we are all familiar from our schooldays, is not enough. Nor is it enough to shine a light into the eye and determine that it is a healthy eye.

An optometric vision examination, particularly of a child, is a rigorous and lengthy procedure. But it is neither painful nor demanding of the patient. Properly prepared for it, a child can find it interesting or even fun.

The Vision Examination

The American Optometric Association describes the vision examination in these terms: a child is not a miniature adult and, therefore, a child's vision examination varies from that given an adult. With a child, the optometric specialist considers visual difficulties in terms of growth factors and stages of physical and mental achievement.

A thorough examination takes from 30 to 60 minutes on the first visit and includes a battery of tests (many of which are like playing games). Specific tests given will vary with each child's individual needs. Besides the review of the child's health history and an exam to confirm the physical health of its eyes, the thorough vision examination includes:

- tests of the child's ability to see sharply and clearly at near and far distances;
- tests to determine refractive status (nearsightedness, farsightedness and focusing problems);
- a check of eye coordination to be certain the eyes work as a team at both near and far distance;
- a test of the ability to change focus easily from near to far and vice versa;
- a check for any indication of crossed-eyes or indications that the child is not using one of its eyes;
- a test of depth perception;
- motor tests to check eye-hand-foot coordination.

The results of all these tests of visual functioning are then compared to an expected developmental level. Where results fall below expected levels, optometric vision care may be recommended.

6

Vision Care: Lenses, Therapy or Both

When a behavioral optometrist examines a patient and finds evidence of a vision imbalance, different courses of action are possible: a. lenses; b. visual training procedures. Often, lenses and visual training are used together.

Lenses. Often, particularly when vision imbalances are minor, lenses are needed only for schoolwork (to take stress off the vision system). *Behavioral optometrists base their lens prescriptions on concepts different from those used by ophthalmologists and general optometrists.*

In general, the latter two groups use lenses only in one way. They prescribe "compensating" lenses which treat symptoms, not causes. For instance, if a child is nearsighted (commonly a symptom of a vision imbalance) compensating lenses can provide 20/20 eyesight. But as the imbalance worsens, as it almost always does, stronger and stronger lenses usually have to be prescribed to maintain 20/20 sight because the vision imbalance is still there.

Since this approach is sight-oriented, the underlying causes of the nearsightedness (or whatever the symptom) are not being treated. The vision system is not being brought into balance (which might eliminate *the need* for these compensating lenses).

The behavioral optometrist uses lenses in various ways:

- *Preventive lenses* — to prevent a problem in the vision system from starting in those diagnosed to be "at risk."
- *Developmental lenses* — to support and nurture an immature vision system while helping it develop normally and help it cope with visual stress.
- *Remedial lenses* — for a specific problem, such as an inability to sustain focusing, until that ability is adequate.

Vision therapy, sometimes called vision training, involves an array of procedures designed to achieve or maintain an optimum balanced and flexibly functioning vision system. It aims to teach the entire vision system to operate at peak efficiency.

A carefully designed program, tailored specifically by the behavioral optometrist to the individual patient, can:

- help prevent the development of some vision problems such as myopia;
- aid in the proper development of vision abilities;
- enhance the efficiency and comfort of vision functioning and;
- help cure and/or correct existing vision problems.

Good Vision Is Developed Not Inborn

The AOA tells us that vision therapy is based on the fact that vision is *learned*. The ability to see and correctly interpret what is seen does not appear automatically at birth. It develops over a lifetime and is shaped by your experiences and environment.

Some children skip steps in their vision development, sometimes because of illness. Others may not be exposed to the necessary visual experiences or learning opportunities to develop their vision skills adequately.

Modern living puts endless stresses on the vision systems of both children and adults. The impact of hours upon hours of daily TV viewing is a whole new complication, yet to be fully understood in terms of vision development. The school-age child is confronted by reading and writing and other close work repeatedly interrupted by demands to shift focus to a teacher or blackboard. An even newer potential problem is the introduction into classrooms of the computer. Lengthy staring into a display terminal screen may cause a child to start having difficulty focusing back and forth between text and screen. These and other stresses can start or worsen a variety of vision imbalances. Eyes may lose their ability to "team." The farsighted and the nearsighted may become more so. And so on.

A program of optometric vision therapy can protect and repair the system. What the behavioral optometrist does is break down the process of vision into various components. Then the problem areas are treated by reeducating, reinforcing or developing specific vision skills such as:

- clearness of vision at near and far distances
- eye movement skills
- eye focusing skills
- eye aiming skills
- eye-hand coordination
- visual perception, identification and memory

You may consider that all these skills are your natural inheritance. The fact is, from infancy, they must all be enhanced through experience and learning. Most people use them well enough to get along (but often, not as well as they might). A substantial percentage of the population does not learn one or another of these skills—or, worse, are deficient in a number of them.

This is where optometric vision therapy comes in. The behavioral optometrist prescribes a program of visual tasks; they are performed in the optometrist's office, although many are also assigned as home therapy.

The tasks vary widely, depending on the individual's special needs. Some, such as walking on a balance beam or jumping on a trampoline, will seem like play to a child. Others make use of equipment that is space age in its sophistication. The repetition of these visual tasks is aimed at improving vision by improving the integration of all the sensory motor activities with vision at the helm. Behavioral optometry works to enhance visual monitoring ability, visualization skills and visual perceptual abilities, among others.

7

Does Optometric Vision Therapy Really Work?

With optometric vision therapy, behavioral optometrists are getting at the root causes of vision imbalances. They're not just treating symptoms. Optometric vision therapy, according to professional organizations like the AOA, the College of Optometrists in Vision Development and the Optometric Extension Program Foundation, is a treatment program designed to teach the entire vision system to operate at peak efficiency. Based on the fact that vision is primarily a *learned process* that begins at birth, optometric vision therapy is used to help persons learn, relearn or reinforce specific vision skills more efficiently.

The procedures may begin by breaking the bad visual habits that a child has developed—habits that have *taught* the eyes to work separately rather than together. Then they *teach* the child how to use its eyes as a team—moving step by step through all the learning stages that a child should go through to achieve normal eye teaming. (With most children, Nature has already done all this, but sometimes Nature needs a little help.) The process can take a couple of months or a year, depending on the severity of the imbalance.

Dr. Richard S. Kavner and Lorraine Dusky, in their book *Total Vision*, published in 1978, say it has been found that 75 percent of people with crossed-eyes and 85 percent of children with vision-related learning disabilities can be helped by optometric vision therapy.

Drs. Nathan Flax and Robert H. Duckman, in the *Journal of the American Optometric Association* for December 1978, cite a number of studies on the effects of optometric vision training. They cite five studies involving 439 persons who underwent optometric vision therapy for crossed-eyes. Seventy-six percent attained normal two-eyed vision and 86 percent achieved straight eyes. The remainder experienced some degree of improved vision and/or straightening of the eyes.

Another study, which followed up on persons in an earlier study, confirmed that results achieved with vision therapy are long-term, not short-term. Of 81 patients who had been successfully treated for crossed-eyes with vision therapy three to seven years earlier, 96 percent still had straight eyes and 89 percent had normal two-eyed vision.

Drs. Martin H. Birnbaum, Kenneth Koslowe and Robert Sanet, in the *American Journal of Optometry & Physiological Optics* for May 1977, review 23 studies involving more than 1,100 persons whose lazy eye condition was treated with vision therapy. More than 50 percent improved their visual acuity by four lines on the eyechart, or better. More than 33 percent achieved 20/30 acuity or better.

The evidence is abundant. Take, for instance, our often maligned "learning disabled" children. Drs. Robert M. Wold, John R. Pierce and Joan Keddington, in the *Journal of the American Optometric Association* for September 1978, find that the effectiveness of vision therapy was dramatically demonstrated in a 1978 study of 100 learning disabled patients. Although 99 percent of them had passed a routine vision screening for eyesight, *all* had difficulties in one or more areas of vision.

Thirty-nine percent lacked good eye-focusing skills; 96 percent could not change their eye focus easily from near to far and back; 75 percent had difficulty using their eyes together as a team; 94 percent had problems with eye movement skills; and 91 percent lacked good eye-aiming skills. After vision therapy, 80 percent had good eye-focusing skills; 75 percent could change their eye focus easily from near to far and back; 86 percent could use their eyes together as a team; 96 percent improved their eye movement skills; and 75 percent sharpened their eye-aiming skills.

Optometric Vision Therapy for Juvenile Delinquents The AOA tells us that optometric studies have found that learning-related vision problems are a strong contributing factor to juvenile delinquency. They add that, once the underlying vision problems are corrected, delinquents can be on the road to becoming productive members of society. To cite two studies among many that support these findings:

1. In 1982, a 21-month study of 914 juvenile delinquents by Dr. Stanley Kaseno, an optometric specialist in California, showed that nearly nine out of ten youths examined had some kind of vision problem. The only approach to health care that the county had not previously involved in their treatment of these children was behavioral optometry. Lenses to fit the vision needs were prescribed and, once optometric vision training was completed, two significant changes were noted: grades improved and the reading level of the group went from 5th grade to 8.5 grade level. The figures for rearrest went from 50–60 percent down to 9–10 percent. (OEP *News*, July 1982.)

2. In a 1977 Virginia study of 79 male and female juvenile delinquents with diagnosed vision-related learning disabilities, those given specific help, including vision therapy, were roughly six times less likely to come back into the court system. (*Journal of Learning Disabilities*, April 1978.)

Training for Athletes

Even the finest athletes, of all ages, have used optometric vision training to sharpen their skills. Quick reaction time, fast, accurate judgement on distances and objects in motion, sharp, clear images, the perception of the athlete's body attitude and its position in space related to other bodies and objects around it—all these are necessary to superior athletic performance. And they all depend on a good, balanced vision system. Behavior is reaction to information from the vision system.

One optometric study reported in the *AOA News* for September 1, 1979, that even among U.S. Olympic contenders approximately 60 percent could sharpen their competitive performance by improving their vision skills. In fact, optometric vision training played a part in helping both the U.S. men's and U.S. women's volleyball teams to their respective gold and bronze medals in the 1984 Olympics. Many professional sports teams have learned the lesson, too, including the New York Knicks, New York Islanders, New York Yankees,

Kansas City Royals, Dallas Cowboys, Chicago Black Hawks and the San Francisco 49ers among others.

A child who does poorly at sports is often simply a victim of vision problems. Since this kind of failure can affect the child's acceptance by its peers, it can warp relationships and lead to negative self-images. It can lead to a lifetime avoidance of physical activity.

It's a shame to let it happen when help is so readily at hand.

Not a Magic Cure-All

A clarification here is useful. No one health therapy can help everyone. Optometric vision care does not help *all* children with learning and behavior problems; it usually helps those with vision-related learning problems.

A wealth of reliable studies—a sample of which you have just read—document the positive results of optometric vision care. If you are interested in delving more deeply into the subject, a recent three-part paper by Irwin Suchoff, O.D., former Dean of the College of Optometry of State University of New York, and Timothy Petito, O.D., is a definitive bibliography of such research. Part I of the Suchoff, Petito paper, "The Efficacy of Visual Therapy: Accommodative Disorders and Non-Strabismic Anomoties of Binocular Vision," will be published in the *Journal of the American Optometric Association* of early 1986. It is an invaluable reference for consumers whose insurance companies or physicians are interested in current, qualified research on the subject.

8

Repairing the Damage— The Team Approach

When you help youngsters with behavior or learning difficulties develop efficient vision systems, that's usually only the *first* step along the way to helping them develop fully productive and competitive lives. Frequently, these children have not developed efficient skills in reading and writing. They are behind their grade level in most studies. Proper study habits are foreign to them. They often have mild to severe emotional problems, which may range from feelings of unworthiness to rebellious rage.

Fixing the cause of all these problems is one thing. Repairing the damage is another. Often, the repairs call for a team approach. In addition to the behavioral optometrist providing vison therapy, a team can include experts in such fields as education, psychology, nutrition and child development.

All fifteen of the nation's colleges of optometry offer courses in vision training—most have clinics where various types of optometric vision care are available. A number of institutions such as the SUNY College of Optometry, the Illinois College of Optometry, the Eye Institute at the Pennsylvania College of Optometry and Southern California College of Optometry place a strong emphasis on the value of team work. So does Connecticut's internationally celebrated Gesell Institute of Human Development.

Vision and Behavior: An Unbreakable Link

Many names stand out among the leaders of behavioral optometry. From the early pioneers such as Drs. Alexander, Brock, Getman, McCoy and Macdonald to the modern practitioners such as Drs. Apell, Flax, Francke, Forrest, Greenspan, Sherman, Solan, Streff and Wachs, their contributions have been invaluable in forging this remarkable discipline. Yet, there is one individual who seems to tower over the rest; A. M. Skeffington, O.D., D.O.S. is generally regarded as the "father" of behavioral optometry.

In the 1920s, Skeffington began to question what could be done for vision imbalances beyond the simple prescribing of lenses to wear. His creative mind reached out beyond the boundaries of his own field of optometry to involve authorities from other disciplines as diverse as biology, physiology, psychology, neurology, physics and education. From 1928, Skeffington was the mainspring of the Optometric Extension Program for forty years. Now called the Optometric Extension Program Foundation, this was the first organization to develop a wide variety of continuing education courses for its members and to publish education and information pamphlets for the public.

Arnold Gesell, M.D., for whom the Gesell Institute is named, was another of the early investigators who helped establish the foundations for behavioral optometry in the 1930s. Dr. Gesell, widely regarded as one of the world's leading pediatric psychologists, and a specialist in child development, studied vision for almost a decade with a team of experts. The result was the landmark book, *Vision and Its Development in Infant and Child.*

Over the decades, the critical connection between vision and behavior has been painstakingly established. Gradually, the precepts of a revolutionary new health therapy have been developed:

- vision problems may trigger or aggravate learning or behavior problems;
- vision can be trained;
- when vision is treated by optometric specialists, learning and behavior may also change and improve.

Warning: The Great Debate
Yet Insurance Pays And Nader Agrees

Behavioral optometry is a specialty. It is practiced by about 12 percent of the 24,000 doctors of optometry, who have pursued the necessary extra training. On the other hand, the average ophthalmologist, family doctor, pediatrician or child psychologist usually knows little or nothing about behavioral optometry because their colleges do not offer courses in it. Many of them, in all good faith, condemn the idea.

Be warned. You will find a number of otherwise reliable advisors pooh-poohing behavioral optometry. But, the large insurance companies don't. Ralph Nader doesn't. Luci Johnson doesn't. The Connecticut State Police don't. Its use by law enforcement officers is supported in a landmark court decision in 1985. A roll call of professional athletes doesn't.

What does all this prove? Major health insurance companies such as Aetna and Blue Cross/Blue Shield only pay for health care that they have investigated and found sound and necessary. Their coverage includes optometric vision care.

Ralph Nader does not lightly endorse *anything*. But he has endorsed optometric vision therapy in the strongest terms. (The New England Council of Optometrists Public Health Symposium, March 16, 1980.)

Of many examples, one will suffice: an article on optometric vision care in the *Wall Street Journal* of May 29, 1985, quoted Aetna Life & Casualty Company: "We're convinced of its value." The company has offered coverage for optometric vision therapy for "at least a decade." *Why?* Indisputable evidence has established its value.

Look at the back of this handbook for a selection of the reputable scientific studies that led Aetna Life (and other insurance companies) to such a decision; note the professional journals which published them. You'll also find titles of some of the many pamphlets published by the various professional organizations. A well-documented consumer's guide to behavioral optometry is *Seeing Eye to I: The Eye-Brain-Behavior Connection*, by Drs. Edelman and Forkiotis and Hazel Richmond Dawkins, who collaborated on this handbook.

So don't be dissuaded by an advisor who has not looked as deeply into the question of behavioral optometric vision care as Aetna. Or Nader.

9

A Home Guide
for Infant Vision Development

Most babies are born with healthy eyes, free from disease and vision problems. Learning to *use* these eyes is one of the critical first steps in a newborn's development.

Since infants spend a large part of their time learning to see, parents of new babies will be glad to read there's a lot they can do to help infants develop healthy vision systems.

Whether it's the presence of bright wallpaper, the frequent repositioning of the crib or a colorful mobile to provide variety and movement, the points are simple and effective. Our source is the American Optometric Association's background paper on infant's vision and the guidelines developed over many years by the Infant's Vision Clinic at SUNY, in New York City, under the direction of Elliott Forrest, O.D.

> *Early Visual Stimulation.* Keep a dim light burning in the nursery at night so the infant will have something to look at when it wakens.

> Move the crib regularly, as well as the baby's position in the crib so that light will stimulate each eye. Use clear bumper guards so vision is not obstructed.

> Approach, change, feed and even play with the baby from different positions. Talk to your baby as you move around the room, this gives the infant a moving object to follow. During the day, place the child in different rooms so that new sights, objects, patterns and different light will stimulate the vision system.

> For the first two months, keep a bright mobile dangling outside the crib to provide variety and movement. At about eight weeks, move the mobile over the crib so the baby can touch it. This permits reinforcement of tactual and visual information.

Hand-Eye Coordination. Play peek-a-boo by holding the baby's hands before its face; play patty-cake.

Provide blocks, rattles, balls and other toys for the baby to touch, bang and throw. Use objects large enough so they can't be swallowed. As the child gets older, make available toys (including pots and pans) to stack, nest, build, string, toss, push, pull, pound, take apart and put together. Clay or play dough, puzzles, tracing and coloring are also good.

General Visual-Motor Coordination. Give the child freedom to explore the house. Avoid the restraints of a playpen, crib and high chair when they are not required. Let the child move around as much as possible.

Encourage the child to wiggle, roll, crawl and creep. This helps to coordinate the two sides of the body more efficiently, an ability that is reflected in the coordination of the two eyes. Parents, therefore, should not encourage their babies to walk before they have done much crawling and creeping. Set up an obstacle course of boxes, chairs and tables so that the child can creep under, over and between objects.

When the child can walk, encourage the use of a wheelbarrow or some other push-and-balance toy. Encourage the child to run, jump, balance, hop and climb.

To Match Vision With the Other Sensory-Motor Systems. Whenever possible, talk and play with the child. Tell stories and sing songs together.

Offer different objects and have the child tell which is heavier, lighter, noisier, when dropped.

These are some of the ways you can help get your child's vision system off to a healthy start. It cannot be repeated often enough: the child has to *learn to see.* We are not born with *sophisticated* visual abilities.

Adults can depend on vision alone to discriminate and understand the size, shape, texture and weight of objects. Infants need help to understand this type of information. They are dependent in the learning process on touching, feeling, squeezing—tactile evidence that allows them to confirm what their vision notes.

As children grow, they will start to base their judgments of texture, shape, size and weight of objects on visual assessment alone. The sight of a ball will trigger their memories of how it feels and what it weighs without the need for tactile evidence that was necessary earlier.

But in the early stages, the infant's vision system must be carefully nurtured for balanced development.

Infant Vision Should Be Examined, Too

Perhaps the most important safeguard recommended by the AOA is that unless signs of problems occur earlier, a child's first thorough vision exam should be given by the time your child is three. The doctor of optometry who specializes in behavioral, developmental or functional optometry is best qualified to handle this exam.

This exam will cover more than simply determining that the child's eyes are healthy, with the ability to rate well, even as high as 20/20 on the eyechart. It will examine the total vision system to make sure that it is in balance and functioning efficiently and at the appropriate level for a three-year-old. The exam should be repeated again before the youngster enters school and annually thereafter until adulthood.

10

How to Find Help

If you are looking for a doctor of behavioral optometry in your area, the most direct source of information might well be your local general optometrist, who can usually give you the name of a colleague who specializes in behavioral vision care. You can also contact either the College of Optometrists in Vision Development, the Optometric Extension Program Foundation, the Gesell Institute's Department of Vision or the colleges of optometry—addresses are all in the next few pages.

If you have a child who has learning or behavior problems and hasn't yet had a behavioral optometric vision exam, why not have one done promptly? It might well reveal a vision imbalance that has been missed by conventional optometric and ophthalmological examinations and which could be corrected with the proper treatment.

Don't hesitate to phone to discuss your needs. Ask how long an exam usually takes. You cannot have a thorough behavioral vision exam in less than 30 minutes; often it takes 45–60 minutes. Dr. Richard Apell, Director of Gesell's Department of Vision, says that at the Institute they often need up to 90 minutes because many of the patients who come there have severe learning problems and more than 30 visual skills that are important to learning have to be tested. Make sure you receive a yes answer to each of the following questions before you make an appointment.

1. Do you make a full series of nearpoint vision tests?
2. Do you make work- or school-related visual perception tests?
3. Do you provide full vision care and visual training in your office or will you refer me to a colleague if needed?

College Clinics Many of the nation's 15 colleges of optometry have clinics that offer various types of vision care. Most also have faculty who have private practices. Once again, be sure to ask for the names of those who specialize in *behavioral, functional or developmental* optometric vision care.

The Gesell Institute, the Optometric Extension Program Foundation, the American Optometric Association and the College of Optometrists in Vision Development all have lists of optometrists who specialize in this health care. Call or write to them and they will send you details on practitioners in your area. Addresses for these organizations follow.

A number of centers around the country offer behavioral optometric and psycho-educational diagnoses and therapy geared either to slow learners or the learning disabled. One is the Learning & Development Center in Philadelphia, Pennsylvania, of which Martin Kane, O.D., is the Director. Another, the Learning Center, directed by Al Sutton, O.D., is in Miami Beach, Florida. Harry Wachs, O.D., is Director of The Reading Center, George Washington University, Washington, D.C. Dr. Wachs specializes in a Piagetian approach to learning-related problems.

A variety of research projects, some involving school systems, are going on around the country. One, initially sponsored by OEPF, is directed by John Streff, O.D., of the Noel Center, Lancaster, Ohio. The Gesell Institute has another in a school system in Connecticut.

If you have difficulty finding addresses for clinics, centers or practitioners, one of the professional groups whose names and addresses follow may be able to help, but doublecheck that practitioners actually specialize in behavioral optometry by asking questions like those previously mentioned.

Professional Organizations

The American Academy of Optometry was founded in 1922 with the expressed purpose of fostering the continued advancement of the education and knowledge of practicing optometrists. The Academy publishes a monthly journal, the *American Journal of Optometry and Physiological Optics*. In addition, it publishes educational articles and textbooks. The Academy also holds annual educational forums, offers postgraduate courses and encourages research and scientific investigations in optometry and related fields. The Academy has a strict code of ethics and rigid standards of membership. Although the next two organizations, AOA and OEPF, might give the most prompt help, you can contact:

The American Academy of Optometry
Attn: Chairman of the Diplomate in
Binocular Vision & Perception
118 North Oak St., Owatonna, MN 55060

The American Optometric Association (AOA) represents more than 24,000 doctors of optometry and students of optometry. Founded in 1898, the AOA is a federation of local associations representing zones, states and the District of Columbia. A majority of practicing optometrists in the U.S. are members. The AOA publishes *The Journal of the American Optometric Association, AOA News* and a helpful selection of informative booklets for consumers and writers. You will notice that much of the material in this handbook refers to the AOA as its source. AOA publications cover a broad spectrum of optometry, from material on the nurturing of infants' vision to vision development for schoolage children to sports vision and advice on contact lenses.

You can get these publications by outlining your needs and sending them to:

The American Optometric Association
Communications Division
243 North Lindbergh Blvd., St. Louis, MO 63141

The Optometric Extension Program Foundation (OEPF) is international in scope. Founded in 1928, it is the principal provider of postgraduate education to optometrists and was the first organization to develop a wide variety of continuing education courses for optometrists and to publish pamphlets for the general consumer. Among their most popular publications are:

When a Bright Child Has Trouble Reading: Learning Problems

Learning Lenses in Beginning Grades: Stress-relieving Lenses

Psychological Effects of Visual Training

The Optometric Extension Program Foundation
2912 South Daimler St., Santa Ana, CA 92705

The Gesell Institute for Human Development has roots that go back to 1911 when Arnold Gesell, M.D., founded his clinic for child study at Yale University. Today, the Institute is a private, nonprofit foundation for research, service and teaching in the field of human development. Its Department of Vision puts particular emphasis on research defining the critical relationship between vision and behavior.

The Gesell clinic offers optometric vision care for youngsters and stresses the value of a team approach to its service. Many behavioral optometrists have taken their graduate training at Gesell, which also offers workshops and lectures for the general public. For a list of Gesell Institute graduates, write or call:

The Gesell Institute of Human Development
310 Prospect St., New Haven, CT 16511

The College of Optometrists in Vision Development (COVD) is a certifying body for practitioners of comprehensive functional eye care. Now an international organization, COVD was created in 1970 by a merger of other behavioral optometric groups from around the country.

The COVD works with other professional organizations such as the AOA, the OEPF and the American Optometric Student Association among many who are concerned with providing maximum care for the public. They cooperate with the National Association for Children With Learning Disabilities, government agencies and with many non-optometric groups who are interested in related problems.

COVD publishes the *Journal of Optometric Vision Development*. In addition, COVD has created dozens of educational pamphlets for optometrists, professionals in health care, parents and educators.

The College of Optometrists in Vision Development
353 H St., Suite C, Chula Vista, CA 92010

Volunteers for Vision, Inc. This Texas-based organization was created in 1965 under the Community Action Program and Project Head Start. Its purpose is to instruct volunteers on how to conduct screening programs for 3–6 year olds. These programs may be at preschool centers, parochial schools, public schools, or federally sponsored day care centers, wherever there is concern for the visual welfare of children. The screening programs are never a substitue for the complete visual examination that can be made only by a professional in the field of vision care, but Volunteers for Vision, Inc., offers an invaluable service which has helped many. Their booklet, the *Manual of Instructions, A Guide for the Vision Screening of Children* is available from Volunteers for Vision, Inc., P.O. Box 2211, Austin, Texas 78768, and the organization's secretary is glad to discuss the developing of a screening program with educational institutions.

Recommended Reading The general reader doesn't have a wide choice of books about behavioral optometry. Arnold Gesell's volume, *Vision—Its Development in Infant and Child*, is the fruit of almost a decade of intensive work by a team of experts. It paved the way for probing research into the connection between behavior and vision by the Gesell Institute's Department of Vision, but although clearly written, it is aimed at professionals in the fields of psychology, optometry and education. First published in 1940, *Vision* does not have any information on the subsequent development and practice of behavioral optometry; nevertheless, it is an illuminating introduction to the origins of behavioral optometry.

In contrast, *Total Vision* by Richard Kavner, O.D., and Lorraine Dusky, an exceptionally fine book, is aimed at the general reader and has a wealth of information on behavioral optometry.

Edelman, E., Forkiotis, C., and Richmond Dawkins, H. *Seeing Eye to I, The Eye-Brain-Behavior Connection*. To be published.

Friedman, E., Lulow, K. *Dr. Friedman's Vision Training Program*. New York. Bantam Books, 1983.

Gesell, A., et al. *Vision—Its Development in Infant and Child*. New York. Harper & Row, 1971 (1st Edition 1940).

Getman, G. N. *How to Develop Your Child's Intelligence.* Irvine, California. Research Publications, 1982 (orig. pub. 1958).

Gregory, R. L. *Eye and Brain.* New York. World University Library/McGraw-Hill, 1966.

Hoopes, A. and T. *Eye Power.* New York. Knopf, 1979.

Kavner, R. and Dusky, L. *Total Vision.* New York. A. and W. Publishers, 1979.

Kavner, R. *Your Child's Vision, A Parent's Guide to Seeing, Growing, and Developing.* New York. Simon & Schuster Inc., 1985.

Seiderman, A. and Schneider, S. *The Athletic Eye.* New York. Hearst, 1983.

Solan, H. A., ed. *The Treatment & Management of Children with Learning Disabilities.* Springfield, Illinois. Charles C. Thomas, 1982.

Streff, J. Ames, A. B. and Gillespie, J. *Stop School Failure.* New York. Harper & Row, 1972.

Helpful Periodicals The professional journals such as the *Journal of the American Optometric Association, American Journal of Optometry and Physiological Optics* and the *Journal of Learning Disabilities* all have excellent articles. Your optometrist may have copies which you can borrow, or have your library make an interlibrary loan, if possible, from one of the colleges of optometry.

Most general readers will find the regular feature, "My Most Interesting Case," in *Optometry Times,* fascinating reading even when, as occasionally happens, they are written in technical language.

Perhaps the clearest material for the consumer is that published by the American Optometry Association, particularly AOA's *Optometric Care Advice for Infants and Children News Backgrounder* and *Vision Therapy News Backgrounder,* and the many pamphlets, such as *Spelling: A Visual Skill* and those listed on pp. 41 and 42, from the Optometric Extension Program Foundation and the College of Vision Development. You'll find addresses in the previous section dealing with these organizations. If you are buying in quantity, you can ask for group rates.

Appendix

Colleges of Optometry (by State)

University of Alabama
School of Optometry, The
  Medical Center
University Station
Birmingham, AL 35294

University of California Berkeley
School of Optometry
360 Minor Hall
Berkeley, CA 94720

Southern California College of
  Optometry
2575 Yorba Linda Blvd.
Fullerton, CA 92631–1699

Illinois College of Optometry
3241 South Michigan Avenue
Chicago, IL 60616

Indiana University School of
  Optometry
800 East Atwater Avenue
Bloomington, IN 47401

New England College of
  Optometry
424 Beacon Street
Boston, MA 02115

Ferris State College of Optometry
Big Rapids, MI 49307

University of Missouri, at St.
  Louis
School of Optometry
8001 Natural Bridge Road
St. Louis, MO 63121

The Ohio State University
College of Optometry
338 West 10th Street
Columbus, OH 43210

The College of Optometry
Pacific University
2043 College Way
Forest Grove, OR 97116

Pennsylvania College of
  Optometry
1200 West Godfrey Avenue
Philadelphia, PA 19141

Inter-American University of
  Puerto Rico
School of Optometry
G.P.O. Box 3255
San Juan, PR 00936

State University of New York
State College of Optometry
122 East 25th Street
New York, NY 10010

Southern College of Optometry
1245 Madison Avenue
Memphis, TN 38104

University of Houston
College of Optometry
4901 Calhoun
Houston, TX 77004

Scientific Studies

This small selection is from a wealth of reputable scientific studies which establish the efficiency of behavioral optometric vision care. A full bibliography is in "The Efficacy of Visual Therapy: Accommodative Disorders and Non-Strabismic Anomolies of Binocular Vision," Part I of III, by Drs. I. Suchoff and G. T. Petito, in the *Journal of the American Optometric Association*, in press 1986. Scientific studies are reviewed in the professional journals in "Helpful Periodicals." The *Journal of the College of Vision Development* also publishes bibliographies of studies.

Bachara, G. H., and Zaba, J. N. "Learning Disabilities and Juvenile Delinquency: Beyond the Correlation." *J. Learning Disabilities* 2(4), April 1978.

Birnbaum, M., Koslowe, K., Sanet R. "Success in amblyopia therapy as a function of age: a literature review." *Am. J. Optom. & Physiol. Opt.* 54(4):269–275, 1977.

Ciuffreda, K. J., Kenyon, R. V., Stark, L. "Different rates of functional recovery of eye movements during orthoptic treatment in an adult amblyope. *Invest. Opthal. & Vis. Sci.* 18(2):213–219, 1979.

Ciuffreda, K. J., Goldrich, S. G., Neary, C. "Use of eye movement auditory biofeedback in the control of nystagmus," *Am. J. Optom. & Physiol. Opt.* 59(5):396–409, 1982.

Cooper, J., Selenow, A., Ciuffreda, K. J., Feldman, J., Faverty, J., Hokoda, S., Silver, J. "Reduction of aesthenopia in patients with convergence insufficiency after fusional vergence training." *Am. J. Optom & Physiol. Opt.* 60(12):982–989, 1983.

Daum, K. "The course and effect of visual training on the vergence system." *Am. J. Optom. & Physiol. Opt.* 59(3):223–227, 1982.

Daum, K. "Accommodative insufficiency." *Am. J. Optom. & Physiol. Opt.* 60(5):352–359, 1983.

Flax, N., Duckman, R. "Orthoptic treatment of strabismus." *J. Amer. Optom. Assoc.* 49(12):1353–1360, 1978.

Goldrich, S. "Optometric therapy of divergence excess strabismus. *Am. J. Optom. & Physiol. Optics* 57(1):7–14, 1980.

Goldrich, S. "Oculomotor biofeedback therapy for exotropia." *Am. J. Optom. & Physiol. Optics* 59(4):306–317, 1982.

Hoffman, L., Cohen, A., Feur, G., Klayman, L. "Effectiveness of optometric therapy for strabismus in a private practice." *Am. J. Optom. & Physiol. Opt.* 47(12):990–995, 1970.

Ludiam, W., Kleinman, B. "The long range results of orthoptic treatment of strabismus." *Am. J. Optom. & Physiol. Opt.* 42(11):647–684, 1965.

Peters, H. B. "Vision Care of Children in a Comprehensive Health Program," *J. Am. Opt. Assn.* 37(12), December 1966, updated statistics to 1979.

Selenow, A., Ciuffreda, K. "Vision function recovery during orthoptic therapy in an exotropic amblyope with high unilateral myopia." *Am. J. Optom. & Physiol. Opt.* 60(8):659–666, 1983.

Solan, H. "A Rationale for the Optometric Treatment and Management of Children with Learning Disabilities." *J. Learning Disabilities.* 14(10), December 1981.

Solan, H., Mozlin, R., Rumpf, D. "The Relationship of Perceptual-Motor Development to Learning Readiness in Kindergarten: A Multivariate Analysis." *J. Learn. Disabilities* 18(6), June/July 1985.

Vaegan: "Convergence and divergence show longer and sustained improvements after short isometric exercises." *Am. J. Optom. & Physiol. Opt.* 56(1):22–33, 1979.

Weisz, C. L. "Clinical therapy for accommodative responses: transfer effects on performance." *J. Am. Optom. Assoc.* 50(2):209–214, 1979.

ABOUT THE AUTHORS

Ellis S. Edelman, O.D., received his Doctorate in Optometry from the Pennsylvania College of Optometry and is a graduate of the Gesell Institute's postdoctoral course in behavioral optometry. An Associate of the College of Vision Development and the Optometric Extension Program Foundation, Dr. Edelman specializes in optometric vision care at Newtown Square, Pennsylvania.

Constantine Forkiotis, O.D., was a classmate of Dr. Edelman at both the Pennsylvania College of Optometry and the Gesell Institute. A Fellow of the American Academy of Optometry and the College of Vision Development, Dr. Forkiotis is active in many organizations, including the Connecticut State Board of Education. In private practice, Dr. Forkiotis specializes in optometric vision care in Fairfield, Connecticut.

Hazel Richmond Dawkins is a veteran editor-writer whose career began in London's Fleet Street newspaper world and has since taken her to Paris, Geneva and New York City. She has worked for major publishers including Harper & Row and Chilton. Among the titles for which she is best known are *Sugar Blues* by William Dufty and *Menopause* by Rosetta Reitz. Ms. Dawkins now lives and works in Wayne, Pennsylvania.

The Connecticut State Police have used the behavioral optometric vision programs Dr. Forkiotis developed for them since 1970. A consultant for the U.S. Department of Transportation Research Office and the National Health Traffic Safety Administration for drug-testing detection and the National Standardized Behavioral Sobriety tests, Dr. Forkiotis was invited by the State of Iowa to present an Expert Witness Course to Police Training Officers, State Prosecuting Attorneys, County Attorneys and Behavioral Optometrists in 1985.

For additional copies and group discounts contact:

The Writing Team
210 Poplar Avenue
Wayne, Pa. 19087

REVIEWS OF

The Suddenly Successful Student

"An examination of a learning disabled child without a consultation and treatment by a developmental optometrist is an incomplete examination and treatment. . . . an authoritative publication for parents . . . pediatricians . . . and psychologists. . . ."

Allan Cott, M.D., Psychiatrist, New York City; Attending Gracie Square Hospital.

". . . easy to read, informative and motivating. Valuable to parents and teachers but should also be read by all medical doctors dealing with problem children. . . . should be part of required medical reading."

Dorothea M. Linley, M.D., General Practitioner, Easton, Conn.

". . . the book as a whole is well written and offers clear concise explanations of the problems involved in the diagnosis and subsequent therapy of learning disabilities."

A. A. Heiger, M.D., Pediatric Associates of Cheshire, Conn., Attending Yale–New Haven Hospital, St. Mary's & Waterbury.

"Good, authoritative manuals for parents of children with learning problems are rare. As a psychologist, I value highly what this book succeeds in doing."

F. A. Schwartz, Ph.D., School Psychologist, Philadelphia, Pa., Co-Director, Bustleton Guidance Center.

". . . a welcome publication. Pediatricians often see children whose visual acuity is normal but who suffer significant deficits in the ability to utilize effectively the mechanisms for focussing and holding a fixed position of the eyes on the task at hand. The field of behavioral optometry has much to offer. . . ."

Morris A. Wessel, M.D., Pediatrician, New Haven, Conn. Attending Yale–New Haven & St. Raphael Hospitals

"I have been exposed to the optometric as well as the ophthalmological phases of eyecare and am much interested in this book because I have never seen such a publication which explains just what behavioral optometry is. I refer appropriate patients . . . and in every instance they benefit a great deal."

George DuPont, M.D., Physician & Surgeon of the Eye, Diplomate, American Board of Ophthalmology, Newport Beach, Calif.